Have you ever paused, even for a fleeting moment, to contemplate the vastness of your own mind? Imagine standing at the edge of a great abyss, peering into the depths of something so immense, so intricate, that it defies comprehension. The human mind is one of the most profound and enigmatic realms we can explore, a place where reality and imagination blur, where the known meets the unknown, and where the deepest mysteries of existence lie hidden in plain sight.

To venture into the depths of your mind is to embark on a journey like no other. It is an expedition into a world where every thought, every emotion, and every perception intertwines to create the unique tapestry of your reality. Here, the boundaries of time and space dissolve, and the familiar becomes unfamiliar. What is real? What is illusion? The answers are not always clear, but the exploration itself is where the true adventure lies.

As you dive deeper, you may encounter the subconscious, that vast reservoir of memories, desires, fears, and dreams that shapes your waking life in ways you might never have imagined. It is here that you begin to understand the powerful forces that influence your thoughts and actions, often without your conscious awareness. This hidden dimension of the mind holds the key to understanding not just who you are, but how you perceive and interact with the world around you.

And then, there's the question of reality itself. What is reality? Is it the tangible world you can see, touch, and measure? Or is it something more elusive, something constructed by your mind as it interprets the endless stream of sensory information it receives? As you delve into these questions, you might begin to see reality not as a fixed and objective truth, but as a fluid, ever-changing experience shaped by your perceptions, beliefs, and inner world.

In exploring these mysteries, you're not merely engaging in an intellectual exercise; you are challenging the very essence of what it means to be human. You are questioning the nature of existence, the fabric of reality, and the limitless potential of your own mind. This journey into the depths of consciousness is one of self-discovery, where each revelation brings you closer to understanding the profound connections between your inner world and the outer reality you experience.

So, are you ready to embark on this journey? To unlock the secrets of your mind and, in doing so, perhaps glimpse the true nature of reality itself? The path ahead may be uncertain, filled with challenges and questions that have no easy answers, but it is a path that promises to transform the way you see yourself and the world around you.

Welcome to the adventure of a lifetime, where the most extraordinary discoveries are not found in the distant corners of the universe, but within the infinite depths of your own mind.

Imagine a world where the power of your subconscious mind shapes every aspect of your life. Daily, your thoughts and mental images influence your style and determine your future. This is your key to unlocking that power.

Have you ever wondered why one person is joyful and prosperous while another is sorrowful and struggling? Why one is brimming with confidence and success while another languishes in fear and doubt? These questions are at the heart of this book.

I wrote this book to demystify the incredible influence of your mind in simple, everyday language. You'll discover profound truths about your mind and life that can transform confusion into clarity, misery into joy, and failure into success.

In these pages, you'll learn how to tap into a miraculous power within you—one that can heal emotional wounds, dissolve physical ailments, and set you free from limitations. It's about unleashing the boundless potential of your subconscious mind, the very force that governs your existence.

Over a decade ago, I witnessed firsthand the astonishing healing capabilities of my subconscious mind, curing what medical science called incurable. I share this technique with you, confident that it can unleash similar healing in your life.

Join me to discover how scientific prayer—a synergy of your conscious and subconscious minds—can bring about profound changes. You hold the key to unlocking the miraculous healing power within you, transforming your life into a testament of freedom, happiness, and peace of mind.

During a conversation with a dear doctor friend, I had a revelation: the same creative intelligence that designed my organs shaped my body, and started my heart also possesses the power to heal its own creation. The ancient proverb says, "The doctor dresses the wound, but God heals it." Wonders truly happen when you pray effectively, aligning your conscious and subconscious minds in harmony. This is what I refer to as scientific prayer—an intentional and focused interaction of the mind, aimed at a specific purpose.

I encourage you to read this book multiple times. Each chapter reveals how this extraordinary power works and teaches you how to access the wisdom and inspiration that lie within your subconscious mind. Everyone prays, but do you know how to pray effectively? When was the last time you prayed—not just in an emergency, or when facing danger, illness, or the shadow of death—but as part of your daily life?

Prayers are said for countless reasons. Open any newspaper, and you'll read about people praying for a child with a so-called incurable illness, for peace between nations, or for miners trapped in a flooded shaft. The big answers to prayers often make the news, serving as powerful testimonies to the effectiveness of prayer. But what about the simple prayers of children, the daily grace before meals, and the quiet devotions of those seeking a connection with the divine?

I've personally experienced the power of prayer, and I've spoken with many who have witnessed its effects. What sets this book apart is its practical, down-to-earth approach. It offers simple techniques and formulas that you can easily incorporate into your daily life. These methods have been used by men and women around the world. Recently, over a thousand people from various religious backgrounds attended a special class in Los Angeles where they explored the key concepts presented in this book.

In these pages, you'll discover why so many people have asked me, "Why have I prayed and prayed, but received no answer?" You'll also learn various ways to impress your subconscious mind and receive the guidance you seek. This book is a valuable resource that you can turn to whenever you need help.

Do you believe in something? It's not what a person believes that determines the outcome of their prayer; it's how their subconscious mind reacts to the images or thoughts they hold. This is why people from all religions—whether Buddhists, Christians, Muslims, or Jews—can receive answers to their prayers. It's not about the religion itself, but rather a technique, a method based on understanding what you're doing and why. This knowledge can help you bring all the good things in life into your experience.

Essentially, answered prayer is when your heart's deepest desires come true. Everyone longs for health, happiness, security, peace of mind, and true self-expression, yet many struggle to achieve these goals. A university professor recently confided in me, "I know that if I change, I'll get what I want." This sentiment is shared by people everywhere because we all share the same mind. The miracle-working power of your subconscious mind existed long before you and I were born, before any church or civilization. The eternal truths and principles of life predate all religions.

With these thoughts in mind, I urge you to delve into the next few chapters and embrace this remarkable, magical, life-changing power. It has the potential to heal both mental and physical wounds and to liberate the mind from fear.

Within you lies a treasure trove of infinite potential—a gold mine of boundless intelligence and love that can provide everything you need to live a glorious, joyful, and abundant life. Yet, many remain unaware of this hidden wealth, asleep to the vast reservoir of possibilities within their own subconscious mind.

Consider the person who is filled with doubt and fear, who hesitates at every opportunity, saying, "I might fail," or "My money could be lost." Such a mindset holds them back, keeping them stuck in place, afraid to take the steps necessary to move forward. But you don't have to be that person. You can become someone who understands the master secret of all time—a secret far more powerful than atomic energy, thermonuclear power, or even interplanetary travel.

So, what is this master secret, and where can it be found? The answer is astonishingly simple: it resides in your subconscious mind, the very place most people overlook. By learning to connect with and release the hidden power within your subconscious, you can unlock more power, wealth, health, happiness, and joy than you ever imagined.

The truth is, you already possess this incredible power. The key is to learn how to use it effectively and understand its workings so that you can apply it to every aspect of your life. This book offers simple steps and techniques to help you access the information and understanding you need. Deep within your subconscious mind lies infinite intelligence and power, waiting to be developed and expressed. As you begin to recognize these possibilities within your deeper mind, they will manifest in the outer world.

Be open-minded and receptive, and the infinite intelligence within your subconscious will guide you to perfect expression and help you find your true place in the world. With the wisdom of your subconscious mind, you can discover the perfect home, attract the right friends, or connect with ideal business partners. It can even bring you financial freedom and the abundance you deserve.

Your subconscious mind is a wellspring of powerful forces—light, love, and beauty—that you have every right to explore. Though invisible, these forces are incredibly strong, capable of providing answers to every problem and revealing the reasons behind every effect. With this power and knowledge, you can move forward with confidence, abundance, joy, and dominion over your life.

When people feel stuck, the power of their subconscious can set them free, restoring them to health, wholeness, and strength. Once liberated, they are free to venture into the world, experiencing happiness, vibrant health, and joyful self-expression. The miraculous healing power of the subconscious can mend a troubled mind, heal a broken heart, and open the prison doors of your mind, releasing you from all material and physical bonds.

This book is your guide to unlocking this immense power within, enabling you to live a life of freedom, joy, and fulfillment.

To make meaningful progress in any area of life, you need a solid working basis—something you can rely on in any situation. Understanding how your subconscious mind works and practicing its powers with confidence is key to achieving the results you desire. The success of this practice depends on how well you grasp these principles and how effectively you apply them to reach your specific goals.

Just as in chemistry, where two atoms of hydrogen combined with one atom of oxygen create water, the principles governing your subconscious mind operate with similar precision. For example, combining one atom of oxygen with one atom of carbon results in carbon monoxide, a poisonous gas. However, if you add another atom of oxygen, you get carbon dioxide, a harmless gas. These principles are consistent across the world of chemical compounds, and they parallel the workings of your mind.

Consider how water always seeks its own level—a universal law that applies everywhere, just as matter expands when heated. These laws are not just limited to the physical world; they also apply to your subconscious mind. The same universal truth holds: whatever you consistently think about in your subconscious mind will eventually manifest in your life as experiences and events.

Your prayers are answered because your subconscious mind operates on principle. Just as electricity flows from a higher potential to a lower potential, your mind works based on the principles of belief. You must have faith in how your mind functions—believing not just in something external, but in the very power of belief itself.

Everything you experience, every event in your life, is a reaction from your subconscious mind to the thoughts you hold. It's not simply about what you believe on the surface; it's about what you believe deep within your mind. When you believe in the eternal truths and principles of life, you will naturally progress forward, upward, and closer to the divine.

By following the advice in this book about the subconscious mind, you will learn to pray scientifically and effectively, both for yourself and others. Your prayers will be answered according to the universal law of action and reaction. Thought is the beginning of action, and the reaction is the response from your subconscious mind that matches the nature of your thoughts. As a result, your mind will be filled with joy, health, peace, and goodwill, and amazing things will begin to unfold in your life.

Though you have only one mind, it operates in two distinct ways. Modern thinkers recognize the line that separates these two functions. The conscious and subconscious, or the objective and subjective, are different in their powers and roles. These terms—conscious and subconscious—are used throughout this book to describe the dual aspects of your mind.

A great way to understand how your mind works is by grasping these concepts and recognizing how each part of your mind contributes to your overall experience. By doing so, you will unlock the full potential of your subconscious and consciously direct it toward creating the life you desire.

The conscious and subconscious minds work together to shape our reality. Imagine your mind as a garden, where your conscious mind is the gardener, planting seeds that will eventually bloom in your life. These seeds are your thoughts, and what you plant in your subconscious mind will grow and manifest in your body, surroundings, and experiences. If you plant seeds of peace, happiness, and prosperity in your conscious mind, and nurture these thoughts with quiet acceptance and repetition, your subconscious mind will help them flourish into a bountiful harvest.

Both good and bad thoughts can take root in your subconscious mind, which is why it's crucial to manage your thoughts carefully. Your subconscious doesn't question the nature of the seeds; it simply nurtures whatever is planted, growing thoughts into experiences. This means that if you harbor negative or harmful thoughts, they will grow and manifest in your life as negative conditions.

Your subconscious mind is incredibly powerful and, when filled with positive, peaceful, and constructive thoughts, it will respond by bringing about favorable conditions, pleasant surroundings, and overall well-being. Understanding this, you can use the power of your subconscious mind to solve problems and achieve your goals by working in harmony with the universal laws of the mind.

Most people live in the "world without," focusing on external circumstances. But true change and creativity come from the "world within"—your inner thoughts, feelings, and images. The external world is a reflection of your inner world, created by the thoughts and beliefs you hold. If you want to change your life, you must first change your thoughts and beliefs. This inner work will eventually be reflected in the conditions and circumstances of your outer life.

Your conscious mind acts as the captain of your ship, directing your life and making decisions. Your subconscious mind is like the crew in the engine room, carrying out the captain's orders without question. If you continually tell yourself, "I can't afford this," your subconscious mind will accept this as true and ensure that you cannot afford the things you desire. On the other hand, if you affirm that you can achieve something, your subconscious will work to make it happen, as illustrated by the example of a young woman who affirmed she could own a beautiful bag she desired and soon received it as a gift.

The subconscious mind is always working, even when you're not aware of it. It carries out orders based on the thoughts you consciously hold and will manifest these thoughts into reality. This is why it's essential to focus on positive, empowering beliefs and to avoid negative self-talk.

Your mind operates on the principle of belief. Whatever you consciously believe and impress upon your subconscious mind will be accepted as true and will manifest in your life. This is the power of faith and expectation, which can bring about profound changes in your life if directed correctly.

By understanding the conscious and subconscious minds and how they interact, you can begin to use this knowledge to create a better life. Instead of letting negative thoughts and beliefs control you, focus on positive, uplifting thoughts that align with your desires. Your subconscious will respond by bringing these desires into reality, leading to a life of health, success, and fulfillment.

. Your subconscious mind doesn't understand jokes; it takes everything you say at face value. This underscores the importance of auto-suggestion.

Auto-suggestion is a practice where you deliberately offer clear and specific suggestions to yourself. Herbert Parkin, in his great book on the subject, illustrates this with a humorous example: A person from New York, visiting Chicago, forgets the time difference and tells a Chicagoan that it's noon, prompting the local to feel hungry even though it isn't lunchtime yet. This demonstrates how the mind can be influenced by suggestions, whether they are accurate or not.

A young singer, for example, faced severe anxiety during auditions. Although she had a wonderful voice, she constantly told herself, "Maybe they won't like me; I'm full of fear and anxiety." Her subconscious mind took these negative suggestions to heart, creating an automatic fear response. However, she overcame this by practicing positive auto-suggestion. She would lock herself in a room three times a day, relax her body, and calmly repeat affirmations like "I sing beautifully," slowly and with feeling. After a week, she was calm and confident, and her next audition was a success.

Similarly, an elderly woman improved her memory by affirming, "My memory is improving in every department. I shall always remember whatever I need to know." Through persistent positive suggestions, she found that her recall abilities strengthened over time.

Another example is a man who struggled with a bad temper. He began to say to himself, "From now on, I will be more cheerful. Joy, happiness, and cheerfulness are my normal states of mind." Over time, these affirmations transformed his demeanor, making him more lovable and understanding.

On the other hand, hetero-suggestion, where someone else suggests to you, can have profound effects, especially when the suggestions are negative. Throughout history, suggestions have been used to control and direct people who don't understand the power of the mind. For instance, a man once visited a fortune-teller who predicted he would die on the next new moon. The man believed this deeply, and the fear it instilled ultimately led to his death, not because of any mystical power, but because his own subconscious mind acted on the suggestion.

This story emphasizes that other people's ideas only have power over you if you accept them. You must consciously choose which thoughts and suggestions to allow into your subconscious mind. If your conscious mind believes something to be true, your subconscious will work to make it a reality.

Consider the example of a college professor who once attended my lectures on the science of mind. He was experiencing turmoil in his life—losing his health, wealth, and friends. I advised him to affirm that his subconscious mind was infinitely wise and was guiding him towards success. He began to repeat positive affirmations, such as, "Infinite Wisdom leads and guides me in all my ways," and soon after, he saw his life transform.

Your subconscious mind is incredibly powerful and will act on whatever thoughts and beliefs you hold. If you consistently feed it positive, life-affirming thoughts, it will bring those thoughts to fruition. However, if you allow negative suggestions to take root, they can block your path to success. The key is to consciously and deliberately choose thoughts that align with the life you wish to create.

Remember, your subconscious mind is always working in your favor, provided you give it the right instructions. Whether it's healing your body, solving problems, or achieving your goals, the power lies within your mind to bring about the changes you desire. So, calm your mind, trust in your subconscious, and allow its wisdom to guide you toward a fulfilling and joyful life.

Your subconscious mind holds incredible power, capable of performing miracles in ways that even the most brilliant minds in the world cannot fully comprehend. It is the source of ideas, the keeper of memories, and the silent force that drives your body's most vital functions. Your subconscious mind is responsible for starting your heartbeat, regulating your blood flow, and managing digestion, absorption, and elimination. It transforms the food you eat into tissue, muscle, bone, and blood, all without any conscious effort on your part. Even the most knowledgeable scientists and doctors cannot fully explain how this process works—yet your subconscious mind handles it effortlessly.

This same power that manages all the essential processes in your body also knows how to solve your most pressing problems. It never sleeps or rests, constantly working behind the scenes to keep you alive and well. There is a magical power within your subconscious that you can tap into by giving it direct instructions, especially before you go to sleep. By doing so, you set in motion the forces within you that can lead to the outcomes you desire.

This inner power is a source of immense strength and wisdom, connecting you to the greater forces of the universe—the very power that makes the sunshine and keeps the planets in orbit. Your deepest goals, hopes, and desires are all rooted in your subconscious mind, which works tirelessly to help you achieve them.

Throughout history, many great minds have tapped into the power of the subconscious to achieve extraordinary feats. William Shakespeare, for example, seemed to know facts and insights beyond the knowledge of his time, undoubtedly drawn from his subconscious mind. The great Greek sculptor Phidias created works of art that embodied beauty, order, balance, and proportion, guided by the visions of his subconscious mind. This same inner force allowed Raphael to paint his Madonnas and Ludwig van Beethoven to compose his timeless symphonies.

In 1955, during a discussion at Wake Forest University in Michigan, a surgeon from Bombay shared a remarkable story about a Scottish surgeon named Dr. James Esdaile, who worked in Bengal before the discovery of ether and other modern anesthetics. Between 1843 and 1846, Dr. Esdaile performed around 400 major surgeries, including amputations, tumor removals, and eye, ear, and throat operations, using only mental anesthesia. Remarkably, the death rate among his patients was extremely low, possibly as low as 2% to 3%. His patients experienced no pain during surgery and, astonishingly, no one died from infections, even though this was before the germ theory of disease was established by Louis Pasteur and Joseph Lister.

The Indian surgeon explained that Dr. Esdaile achieved these results by speaking directly to his patients' subconscious minds, instructing them that no infection or illness would occur. The subconscious minds of his patients accepted these suggestions, leading to their remarkable recovery. This story highlights the astonishing power of the subconscious mind—a power that, more than 120 years ago, allowed a surgeon to achieve miraculous outcomes that still inspire awe today.

When you consider the spiritual and healing powers of your subconscious mind, it is truly breathtaking. This same power resides within you, ready to be harnessed for your well-being and success. By understanding and tapping into the vast potential of your subconscious mind, you can achieve miracles in your own life, just as these great figures of history have done.

When you reflect on the spiritual power of your subconscious mind, it can stop you in your tracks and fill you with awe. This power sees and hears things beyond ordinary perception, unbound by time or space. It can free you from pain and suffering, solve any problem, and do much more. These abilities remind you that you possess power and wisdom that transcend your conscious mind, leaving you amazed by the possibilities.

Your subconscious mind keeps a detailed record of your life, and whatever beliefs, opinions, or thoughts you impress upon it will manifest as facts, situations, and events in your life. What you internalize will eventually be reflected in your external reality. Thoughts and their manifestations are two sides of the same coin. Your conscious mind, composed of thinking cells, sends thoughts to your brain. Once your conscious mind fully accepts a thought, it is transmitted to the solar plexus, often referred to as the brain of your mind, where it takes shape and appears in your experience.

As we've discussed, your subconscious mind acts only on what you impress upon it. It aligns with your decisions or the directives given by your conscious mind, which is why you continuously add to the "Book of Life." Your thoughts shape your reality, echoing the words of Ralph Waldo Emerson: "Man is what he thinks all day long." The subconscious mind, in turn, influences your conscious awareness.

Some believe that your subconscious mind has the power to change the world. William James, the father of American psychology, recognized that your subconscious mind is wiser and more intelligent than you can imagine. It taps into deep, underground streams of knowledge and is governed by the law of life. Whatever you tell your subconscious mind, it will do its utmost to bring into reality. Therefore, it's essential to feed it positive and constructive thoughts.

Many people suffer because they do not understand how their conscious and subconscious minds interact. True health, happiness, peace, and joy come from the harmonious collaboration of these two aspects of your mind. When your conscious and subconscious minds are in harmony, there is no sickness or conflict.

The ancient saying, "As within, so without; as above, so below," encapsulates this principle. What resides in your subconscious mind manifests in your external world. Throughout history, wise men and women like Moses and Isaiah have taught that your conditions, situations, and events reflect your innermost beliefs. The balance between action and feeling, both within your body and in the world around you, is the most fundamental law of life. Nature operates on the principles of action and reaction, rest and motion—forces that must be balanced for unity and harmony to prevail.

You are here to let the life force flow through you in a steady, balanced way. Your thoughts and attitudes shape your experiences. Negative thoughts lead to negative feelings, which, if not released, can manifest as physical ailments like ulcers, heart problems, stress, and worry. Your current health, financial situation, friendships, and social standing are all reflections of who you think you are—what is engraved in your subconscious mind shows up in every aspect of your life.

Negative thoughts are harmful, but they are not innate. By feeding your subconscious mind positive thoughts, you can overwrite negative patterns and create new, healthy ones. Just as the subconscious mind can heal physical ailments like abnormal skin growths, it can also heal emotional and mental wounds.

Over 5 years ago, I read about and helped a friend who experienced the healing power of the subconscious mind firsthand. Faced with a skin cancer that medicine could not cure, I turned to prayer. A clergyman well-versed in psychology explained the deeper meaning of Psalm 139: "In thy book were written all my members, which were continually made when there were none of them." He told me that "book" referred to my subconscious mind, which had created my body and could restore it to health by following the perfect pattern within.

He compared the intelligence in my subconscious to a watchmaker who knows how to repair a malfunctioning watch. Similarly, my subconscious, which had shaped my body, knew how to heal and restore it. But first, I needed to communicate to it my desire for health.

I prayed simply: "The infinite intelligence in my subconscious mind created my body and all its parts. It knows how to heal me. Its wisdom shaped all my organs, tissues, muscles, and bones. This infinite healing presence within me is now transforming every part of my being, making me whole and perfect. I thank the creative intelligence within me for my healing. I know it is happening now. Wonderful are its works." Within three months, my face was completely healed.

This experience showed me that by giving my subconscious mind life-affirming patterns of wholeness, beauty, and perfection, I could eliminate the negative images and thoughts causing my ailment. Nothing appears on your body until it is first conceived in your mind. When you change your mind by filling it with positive thoughts, your body follows suit. This is the foundation of all healing.

As Psalm 139:14 declares, "Wonderful are your works, and my soul knows it very well." Your subconscious mind controls all bodily functions, whether you are awake or asleep. It keeps your heart beating, your lungs breathing, and your blood oxygenated, just as effectively when you're asleep as when you're awake.

Consider the remarkable story of a man whose subconscious mind acted like a film, with his mental picture of healing entrenched through weeks of focused thought. One day, when his phone rang while his wife and nurse were away, he managed to answer it despite it being 12 feet away. This was the moment of his healing. By concentrating on his subconscious mind's healing power, he activated it, enabling himself to walk despite previously believing he couldn't.

This illustrates the profound influence of the subconscious mind. It can be likened to a hidden reservoir of healing power, which many people have believed exists within them for centuries. Historical accounts from diverse cultures suggest that ancient priests and holy men wielded this power, invoking it through prayers, rituals, and various symbols to effect healing. Such practices varied widely—some involved laying on of hands, while others used amulets, talismans, or incantations.

Even today, your subconscious mind is continually at work, regulating essential bodily functions whether you are awake or asleep. For example, your heart beats rhythmically, and your lungs maintain their function without conscious effort. Your subconscious mind also oversees intricate processes like digestion and hormonal secretions. Notably, while you sleep, your body continues vital functions like growing hair and secreting sweat, and many great discoveries have been made in dreams.

However, negative emotions such as worry, anxiety, and sadness can disrupt the natural rhythm of your body's systems. To restore harmony, it's essential to calm your mind and let your subconscious take over in a peaceful and orderly manner. Communicate with your subconscious mind with conviction, and it will respond accordingly, striving to maintain your well-being.

Your subconscious mind is inherently geared to keep you alive and healthy. It manifests protective instincts, such as making you vomit if you ingest something harmful. When you trust in its miraculous power, it works to restore your health.

To harness this power effectively, first understand that your subconscious is always active, operating round the clock regardless of your conscious awareness. Your conscious mind needs to focus on positive, constructive thoughts. By keeping your conscious mind occupied with uplifting expectations, you allow your subconscious to generate beneficial outcomes.

Consider the healing principle observed in the story of a woman from France who regained her sight despite having lifeless optic nerves. This miraculous event, reported by Ruth Cranston in McCall's magazine, underscores how belief and faith in one's subconscious mind can bring about healing. Madame's restoration of sight was not due to external factors but rather the response of her subconscious mind to her faith.

Similarly, in Johannesburg, a Protestant preacher used a technique to visualize perfect health, affirming it with deep relaxation and positive beliefs. This method led to a remarkable recovery from leukemia. Another example involved a man with functional paralysis who visualized himself walking and performing daily activities. His subconscious mind accepted this mental picture and helped restore his health.

Historically, various healing practices involved hypnotic suggestions and rituals to engage the subconscious mind, leading to notable recoveries. These practices reveal that the power of the subconscious mind, when aligned with faith and belief, can effectuate significant changes.

The biblical perspective reinforces this concept. As mentioned in the Bible, "Whatever you pray for, believe that you have received it, and it will be yours." This principle suggests that to manifest your desires, you must fully believe and accept that your wish is already fulfilled. Faith plays a crucial role, as the mind must envision the desired outcome as a reality to bring it into existence. This belief must be deeply ingrained in your subconscious, nurturing it like a seed that will grow into reality.

By focusing your thoughts on positive outcomes and reinforcing them with unwavering faith, you can tap into the creative power of your subconscious mind, making your goals and desires a reality. Just as seeds grow into plants with the right care, your beliefs and expectations shape your life's experiences.

You can harness the creative power of your mind by following these steps. In the world of the subconscious, your thoughts, ideas, plans, and goals become real, much like your physical body parts. The biblical method for achieving this involves eliminating any conditions or events that might suggest failure. By planting a positive idea or goal in your subconscious mind and leaving it undisturbed, it will grow into reality. Faith is crucial here; it's akin to believing that seeds you plant will grow into plants because you trust in the rules of growth and farming.

The Bible emphasizes faith as a way of thinking, a state of mind, and an inner certainty that the thought you accept will manifest in reality. Faith involves trusting in what may seem improbable or impossible to the conscious mind and surrendering to the power of the subconscious. This means setting aside logical skepticism and fully embracing the potential of your subconscious mind to effect change.

Miracles at shrines around the world offer compelling evidence of this principle. In Japan, for example, people visit the famous shrine of the Great Buddha, a 42-foot bronze statue known for its meditative pose. Visitors make offerings, light candles, and express their pleas. One young girl, after praying and making offerings, regained her voice—a miraculous event she attributed to Buddha's intervention. Her faith and ritual created a mental state that allowed her subconscious mind to respond and heal her.

Consider the story of a family member with cancer whose recovery illustrates the power of faith and imagination. His son, believing deeply in the healing power of a relic, fabricated a piece of wood to resemble a sacred artifact. When his father held it, prayed, and went to sleep, his condition improved remarkably. The real healing came from his awakened faith and imagination, not from the actual relic.

This demonstrates a universal healing principle: regardless of the method or tradition, the underlying power is the subconscious mind. Different healing practices—from osteopathy and chiropractic medicine to various religious rituals—are all rooted in this single process. Faith plays a vital role; it triggers the subconscious mind's healing capabilities.

Research into hypnosis shows that the subconscious mind can influence bodily functions significantly. For instance, a person under hypnosis can exhibit symptoms like high fever or chills based solely on suggestions. Similarly, a hypnotic subject can develop allergic reactions or other conditions purely through suggestion, highlighting that the mind's influence extends to physical health.

Remarkable healings also occur through other forms of therapy, such as osteopathy and chiropractic methods, demonstrating the same principle: the subconscious mind as the primary healer. The body's natural healing processes, such as fixing a cut, rely on the subconscious mind's ability to maintain and restore health.

Historical figures like Paracelsus, a Swiss alchemist and surgeon, recognized the power of faith in healing. He asserted that whether faith is placed in a genuine or false object, the results will be the same. This view was echoed by other thinkers who saw the effects of faith and imagination as critical to healing.

In modern times, examples like Dr. Bernheim's experiments with suggestive therapies further illustrate the power of the subconscious mind. By applying simple suggestions, he could induce symptoms or even cause physical changes, reinforcing the idea that the subconscious mind governs our physical state.

The principle remains clear: the subconscious mind is central to all healing. Whether through faith, imagination, or suggestion, the true power lies in how deeply we engage our subconscious beliefs and expectations.

Dear Friends and Family,

As I sit down to write this letter, I find myself overwhelmed with gratitude for each and every one of you. Your unwavering support, encouragement, and belief in me have been nothing short of incredible. Whether it was cheering me on from the sidelines, offering words of wisdom, or simply being there to listen, your presence in my life has made all the difference.

Writing is often seen as a solitary pursuit, but your support has shown me that it truly takes a village. You've celebrated my successes and lifted me up during moments of doubt. Your belief in the bigger picture, in my dreams and aspirations, has been a constant source of motivation.

It's not just about the words on the page; it's about the journey we've taken together. Each of you has played a unique role in shaping who I am as a writer and as a person. Your insights, love, and unwavering support have inspired me to keep pushing forward, even when the path seemed uncertain.

Thank you for believing in me, even when I struggled to believe in myself. Thank you for understanding the sacrifices that come with pursuing a dream. Thank you for your patience, your understanding, and your endless encouragement.

As I continue on this journey, know that I carry each of you in my heart. Your support has not only helped me achieve my goals but has also enriched my life in ways I cannot fully express. I am truly blessed to have such incredible friends and family by my side.

With deepest gratitude and love,

A Prayer of Gratitude

Heavenly Father, Creator of all that is seen and unseen, I come before You with a heart overflowing with gratitude. Words seem inadequate to express the depth of my thankfulness, but I offer them with sincerity, knowing that You understand even the quietest whispers of my soul.

Thank You, Lord, for the breath in my lungs, the beating of my heart, and the life You have graciously bestowed upon me. Every moment I wake is a testament to Your mercy, and every step I take is guided by Your unfathomable wisdom. I am in awe of Your creation—the beauty of the world around me, the intricacies of life, and the wonder of existence. Each sunrise reminds me of Your faithfulness, each starry night of Your infinite majesty.

I thank You for the challenges and trials that have shaped me, for I know that in every difficulty lies a lesson, and in every sorrow, a deeper understanding of Your love. You have been my strength when I was weak, my comfort in times of despair, and my light in the darkest of days. Even when I could not see the path ahead, You were there, guiding me with a love that knows no bounds.

Thank You for the blessings I often take for granted—the warmth of a home, the embrace of loved ones, the food that nourishes my body, and the peace that calms my spirit. I am grateful for the people You have placed in my life, each one a reflection of Your love and a reminder of the community You have woven around me. May they feel Your presence as I do, and may they be blessed abundantly for the kindness and love they have shown me.

Lord, I thank You for Your Word, a source of wisdom, guidance, and comfort. In its pages, I find the strength to persevere, the courage to face my fears, and the reassurance that I am never alone. Your promises are my anchor, and Your truth is my foundation.

As I offer this prayer of thanks, I humbly ask for Your blessings upon all who read these words. May they feel Your love surrounding them, filling their hearts with peace and their lives with joy. May they find strength in Your presence, comfort in Your promises, and hope in the knowledge that You are with them always.

Bless them, Lord, with the abundance of Your grace. Grant them wisdom in their decisions, peace in their hearts, and joy in their journey. May Your light guide their steps, and Your love be a constant reminder of the goodness that comes from walking in Your ways.

Father, I lift up to You all the desires of my heart, spoken and unspoken, knowing that You hear and answer in ways that are beyond my understanding. I trust in Your timing, Your will, and Your infinite goodness.

With every breath, I give You thanks. With every thought, I praise Your name. May my life be a reflection of the gratitude I feel, and may all that I do bring glory to You, the Most High, now and forever.

In Your holy name, I pray.

Amen.

(In Spanish)

¿Alguna vez te has detenido, aunque sea por un breve momento, a contemplar la inmensidad de tu propia mente? Imagina estar al borde de un gran abismo, mirando hacia las profundidades de algo tan inmenso, tan intrincado, que desafía toda comprensión. La mente humana es uno de los reinos más profundos y enigmáticos que podemos explorar, un lugar donde la realidad y la imaginación se mezclan, donde lo conocido se encuentra con lo desconocido, y donde los misterios más profundos de la existencia yacen ocultos a simple vista.

Adentrarse en las profundidades de tu mente es embarcarse en un viaje como ningún otro. Es una expedición a un mundo donde cada pensamiento, cada emoción y cada percepción se entrelazan para crear el tapiz único de tu realidad. Aquí, los límites del tiempo y el espacio se disuelven, y lo familiar se vuelve extraño. ¿Qué es real? ¿Qué es ilusión? Las respuestas no siempre son claras, pero la propia exploración es donde reside la verdadera aventura.

A medida que te sumerges más profundo, puedes encontrarte con el subconsciente, ese vasto reservorio de recuerdos, deseos, miedos y sueños que moldea tu vida despierta de maneras que quizás nunca hayas imaginado. Es aquí donde comienzas a comprender las poderosas fuerzas que influyen en tus pensamientos y acciones, a menudo sin que te des cuenta. Esta dimensión oculta de la mente contiene la clave para entender no solo quién eres, sino cómo percibes e interactúas con el mundo que te rodea.

Y luego está la pregunta de la realidad misma. ¿Qué es la realidad? ¿Es el mundo tangible que puedes ver, tocar y medir? ¿O es algo más elusivo, algo construido por tu mente mientras interpreta el flujo interminable de información sensorial que recibe? Al profundizar en estas preguntas, podrías empezar a ver la realidad no como una verdad fija y objetiva, sino como una experiencia fluida y en constante cambio, moldeada por tus percepciones, creencias y mundo interior.

Al explorar estos misterios, no estás simplemente participando en un ejercicio intelectual; estás desafiando la esencia misma de lo que significa ser humano. Estás cuestionando la naturaleza de la existencia, el tejido de la realidad y el potencial ilimitado de tu propia mente. Este viaje hacia las profundidades de la conciencia es uno de autodescubrimiento, donde cada revelación te acerca a comprender las conexiones profundas entre tu mundo interior y la realidad exterior que experimentas.

Entonces, ¿estás listo para emprender este viaje? ¿Para desbloquear los secretos de tu mente y, al hacerlo, quizás vislumbrar la verdadera naturaleza de la realidad misma? El camino que tienes por delante puede ser incierto, lleno de desafíos y preguntas que no tienen respuestas fáciles, pero es un camino que promete transformar la manera en que te ves a ti mismo y al mundo que te rodea.

Bienvenido a la aventura de tu vida, donde los descubrimientos más extraordinarios no se encuentran en los rincones distantes del universo, sino dentro de las profundidades infinitas de tu propia mente.

Imagina un mundo en el que el poder de tu mente subconsciente moldea cada aspecto de tu vida. Diariamente, tus pensamientos e imágenes mentales influyen en tu estilo y determinan tu futuro. Esta es tu clave para liberar ese poder.

¿Alguna vez te has preguntado por qué una persona es alegre y próspera mientras que otra está triste y luchando? ¿Por qué una rebosa de confianza y éxito mientras que otra languidece en el miedo y la duda? Estas preguntas son la base de este libro.

Escribí este libro para desmitificar la increíble influencia de tu mente en un lenguaje sencillo y cotidiano. Descubrirás verdades profundas sobre tu mente y tu vida que pueden transformar la confusión en claridad, la miseria en alegría y el fracaso en éxito.

En estas páginas, aprenderás a aprovechar un poder milagroso dentro de ti, uno que puede curar heridas emocionales, disolver dolencias físicas y liberarte de limitaciones. Se trata de liberar el potencial ilimitado de tu mente subconsciente, la misma fuerza que gobierna tu existencia.

Hace más de una década, fui testigo de primera mano de las asombrosas capacidades curativas de mi mente subconsciente, que curaba lo que la ciencia médica llamaba incurable. Comparto esta técnica contigo, seguro de que puede desencadenar una curación similar en tu vida.

Únete a mí para descubrir cómo la oración científica, una sinergia de tu mente consciente y subconsciente, puede generar cambios profundos. Tienes la clave para desbloquear el poder curativo milagroso que hay dentro de ti, transformando tu vida en un testimonio de libertad, felicidad y paz mental.

Durante una conversación con un querido amigo médico, tuve una revelación: la misma inteligencia creativa que diseñó mis órganos, dio forma a mi cuerpo y dio origen a mi corazón también posee el poder de curar su propia creación. El antiguo proverbio dice: "El médico cura la herida, pero Dios la cura". Las maravillas suceden realmente cuando oras de manera eficaz, alineando tu mente consciente y subconsciente en armonía. Esto es lo que yo llamo oración científica: una interacción intencional y enfocada de la mente, dirigida a un propósito específico.

Te animo a leer este libro varias veces. Cada capítulo revela cómo funciona este extraordinario poder y te enseña cómo acceder a la sabiduría y la inspiración que se encuentran en tu mente subconsciente. Todo el mundo reza, pero ¿sabes cómo orar de manera eficaz? ¿Cuándo fue la última vez que rezaste, no solo en una emergencia o cuando enfrentabas un peligro, una enfermedad o la sombra de la muerte, sino como parte de tu vida diaria?

Se rezan por innumerables razones. Abre cualquier periódico y leerás sobre personas que rezan por un niño con una enfermedad supuestamente incurable, por la paz entre las naciones o por los mineros atrapados en un pozo inundado. Las grandes respuestas a las oraciones a menudo aparecen en las noticias y sirven como poderosos testimonios de la eficacia de la oración. Pero ¿qué pasa con las sencillas oraciones de los niños, la oración diaria antes de las comidas y las devociones silenciosas de quienes buscan una conexión con lo divino?

He experimentado personalmente el poder de la oración y he hablado con muchas personas que han sido testigos de sus efectos. Lo que distingue a este libro es su enfoque práctico y realista. Ofrece técnicas y fórmulas sencillas que puedes incorporar fácilmente a tu vida diaria. Estos métodos han sido utilizados por hombres y mujeres de todo el mundo. Recientemente, más de mil personas de diversos orígenes religiosos asistieron a una clase especial en Los Ángeles donde exploraron los conceptos clave presentados en este libro.

En estas páginas, descubrirás por qué tanta gente me ha preguntado: "¿Por qué he orado y orado, pero no he recibido respuesta?". También aprenderás varias formas de impresionar a tu mente subconsciente y recibir la guía que buscas. Este libro es un recurso valioso al que puedes recurrir siempre que necesites ayuda.

¿Crees en algo? No es lo que una persona cree lo que determina el resultado de su oración; es cómo su mente subconsciente reacciona a las imágenes o pensamientos que alberga. Por eso, las personas de todas las religiones (budistas, cristianos, musulmanes o judíos) pueden recibir respuestas a sus oraciones. No se trata de la religión en sí, sino de una técnica, un método basado en comprender lo que estás haciendo y por qué. Este conocimiento puede ayudarte a atraer todas las cosas buenas de la vida a tu experiencia.

En esencia, la oración respondida es cuando los deseos más profundos de tu corazón se hacen realidad. Todos anhelamos salud, felicidad, seguridad, paz mental y una verdadera autoexpresión, pero muchos luchan por alcanzar estas metas. Un profesor universitario me dijo recientemente: "Sé que si cambio, conseguiré lo que quiero". Este sentimiento lo comparten personas de todo el mundo porque todos compartimos la misma mente. El poder milagroso de tu mente subconsciente existía mucho antes de que tú y yo naciéramos, antes de cualquier iglesia o civilización. Las verdades y principios eternos de la vida son anteriores a todas las religiones.

Con estos pensamientos en mente, te insto a que profundices en los próximos capítulos y aceptes este extraordinario poder mágico que cambia la vida. Tiene el potencial de curar heridas tanto mentales como físicas y liberar la mente del miedo.

Todo lo que experimentas, cada acontecimiento de tu vida, es una reacción de tu mente subconsciente a los pensamientos que albergas. No se trata simplemente de lo que crees en la superficie, sino de lo que crees en lo más profundo de tu mente. Cuando crees en las verdades y principios eternos de la vida, progresarás naturalmente hacia adelante, hacia arriba y más cerca de lo divino.

Si sigues los consejos de este libro sobre la mente subconsciente, aprenderás a orar de manera científica y eficaz, tanto por ti como por los demás. Tus oraciones serán respondidas de acuerdo con la ley universal de acción y reacción. El pensamiento es el comienzo de la acción y la reacción es la respuesta de tu mente subconsciente que coincide con la naturaleza de tus pensamientos. Como resultado, tu mente se llenará de alegría, salud, paz y buena voluntad, y comenzarán a suceder cosas asombrosas en tu vida.

Aunque tienes una sola mente, esta opera de dos maneras distintas. Los pensadores modernos reconocen la línea que separa estas dos funciones. El consciente y el subconsciente, o el objetivo y el subjetivo, son diferentes en sus poderes y funciones. Estos términos (consciente y subconsciente) se utilizan en todo este libro para describir los aspectos duales de su mente.

Una excelente manera de entender cómo funciona su mente es captar estos conceptos y reconocer cómo cada parte de su mente contribuye a su experiencia general. Al hacerlo, desbloqueará todo el potencial de su subconsciente y lo dirigirá conscientemente hacia la creación de la vida que desea.

La mente consciente y la subconsciente trabajan juntas para dar forma a nuestra realidad. Imagine su mente como un jardín, donde su mente consciente es el jardinero, plantando semillas que eventualmente florecerán en su vida. Estas semillas son sus pensamientos, y lo que plante en su mente subconsciente crecerá y se manifestará en su cuerpo, entorno y experiencias. Si planta semillas de paz, felicidad y prosperidad en su mente consciente, y nutre estos pensamientos con aceptación y repetición silenciosas, su mente subconsciente los ayudará a florecer en una cosecha abundante.

Tanto los pensamientos buenos como los malos pueden echar raíces en su mente subconsciente, por lo que es crucial gestionar sus pensamientos con cuidado. Su subconsciente no cuestiona la naturaleza de las semillas; La mente subconsciente es una mente que simplemente nutre todo lo que se planta, haciendo que los pensamientos se conviertan en experiencias. Esto significa que si albergas pensamientos negativos o dañinos, estos crecerán y se manifestarán en tu vida como condiciones negativas.

Tu mente subconsciente es increíblemente poderosa y, cuando está llena de pensamientos positivos, pacíficos y constructivos, responderá generando condiciones favorables, entornos agradables y bienestar general. Si comprendes esto, puedes usar el poder de tu mente subconsciente para resolver problemas y alcanzar tus metas trabajando en armonía con las leyes universales de la mente.

La mayoría de las personas viven en el "mundo exterior", concentrándose en las circunstancias externas. Pero el verdadero cambio y la creatividad provienen del "mundo interior": tus pensamientos, sentimientos e imágenes internos. El mundo externo es un reflejo de tu mundo interior, creado por los pensamientos y creencias que tienes. Si quieres cambiar tu vida, primero debes cambiar tus pensamientos y creencias. Este trabajo interno eventualmente se reflejará en las condiciones y circunstancias de tu vida exterior.

Tu mente consciente actúa como el capitán de tu barco, dirigiendo tu vida y tomando decisiones. Tu mente subconsciente es como la tripulación en la sala de máquinas, que cumple las órdenes del capitán sin cuestionarlas. Si te dices continuamente a ti mismo: "No puedo permitirme esto", tu mente subconsciente lo aceptará como cierto y se asegurará de que no puedas permitirte las cosas que deseas. Por otro lado, si afirmas que puedes lograr algo, tu subconsciente trabajará para que eso suceda, como lo ilustra el ejemplo de una joven que afirmó que podía tener un hermoso bolso que deseaba y pronto lo recibió como regalo.Spanish)

Como hemos comentado, tu mente subconsciente actúa sólo en función de lo que le imprimes. Se alinea con tus decisiones o con las directivas que te da tu mente consciente, por eso continuamente añades cosas al "Libro de la Vida". Tus pensamientos dan forma a tu realidad, haciendo eco de las palabras de Ralph Waldo Emerson: "El hombre es lo que piensa todo el día". La mente subconsciente, a su vez, influye en tu conciencia.

Algunos creen que tu mente subconsciente tiene el poder de cambiar el mundo. William James, el padre de la psicología americana, reconoció que tu mente subconsciente es más sabia e inteligente de lo que puedas imaginar. Se nutre de corrientes profundas y subterráneas de conocimiento y se rige por la ley de la vida. Cualquier cosa que le digas a tu mente subconsciente, ella hará todo lo posible por convertirla en realidad. Por lo tanto, es esencial alimentarla con pensamientos positivos y constructivos.

Muchas personas sufren porque no entienden cómo interactúan su mente consciente y su mente subconsciente. La verdadera salud, felicidad, paz y alegría provienen de la colaboración armoniosa de estos dos aspectos de tu mente. Cuando tu mente consciente y tu mente subconsciente están en armonía, no hay enfermedad ni conflicto.

El antiguo dicho, "Como es adentro, es afuera; como es arriba, es abajo", resume este principio. Lo que reside en tu mente subconsciente se manifiesta en tu mundo externo. A lo largo de la historia, hombres y mujeres sabios como Moisés e Isaías han enseñado que tus condiciones, situaciones y eventos reflejan tus creencias más íntimas. El equilibrio entre acción y sentimiento, tanto dentro de tu cuerpo como en el mundo que te rodea, es la ley más fundamental de la vida. La naturaleza opera según los principios de acción y reacción, descanso y movimiento, fuerzas que deben equilibrarse para que prevalezcan la unidad y la armonía.

Estás aquí para dejar que la fuerza vital fluya a través de ti de una manera constante y equilibrada. Tus pensamientos y actitudes dan forma a tus experiencias. Los pensamientos negativos conducen a sentimientos negativos, que, si no se liberan, pueden manifestarse como dolencias físicas como úlceras, problemas cardíacos, estrés y preocupación. Tu salud actual, tu situación financiera, tus amistades y tu posición social son todos reflejos de quién crees que eres: lo que está grabado en tu mente subconsciente se refleja en cada aspecto de tu vida.

Los pensamientos negativos son dañinos, pero no son innatos. Si alimentas tu mente subconsciente con pensamientos positivos, puedes sobrescribir patrones negativos y crear otros nuevos y saludables. Así como la mente subconsciente puede curar dolencias físicas como crecimientos anormales en la piel, también puede curar heridas emocionales y mentales.

Hace más de 5 años, leí y ayudé a un amigo que experimentó el poder curativo de la mente subconsciente de primera mano. Ante un cáncer de piel que la medicina no podía curar, recurrí a la oración. Un clérigo muy versado en psicología me explicó el significado más profundo del Salmo 139: "En tu libro estaban escritos todos mis miembros, que fueron creados continuamente cuando no existía ninguno de ellos". Me dijo que "libro" se refería a mi mente subconsciente, que había creado mi cuerpo y podía restaurarlo a la salud siguiendo el patrón perfecto que había dentro de mí.

Comparó la inteligencia de mi subconsciente con un relojero que sabe reparar un reloj que no funciona. De la misma manera, mi subconsciente, que había moldeado mi cuerpo, sabía cómo sanarlo y restaurarlo. Pero primero, necesitaba comunicarle mi deseo de salud.

Oré simplemente: "La inteligencia infinita de mi mente subconsciente creó mi cuerpo y todas sus partes. Sabe cómo sanarme. Su sabiduría moldeó todos mis órganos, tejidos, músculos y huesos. Esta infinita presencia sanadora dentro de mí ahora está transformando cada parte de mi ser, haciéndome completo y perfecto. Agradezco a la inteligencia creativa dentro de mí por mi curación. Sé que está sucediendo ahora. Maravillosas son sus obras". En tres meses, mi rostro estaba completamente curado.

Esta experiencia me mostró que al darle a mi mente subconsciente patrones de afirmación de vida de plenitud, belleza y perfección, podía eliminar las imágenes y pensamientos negativos que causaban mi dolencia. Nada aparece en tu cuerpo hasta que primero es concebido en tu mente. Cuando cambias tu mente llenándola de pensamientos positivos, tu cuerpo hace lo mismo. Esta es la base de toda curación.

Como declara el Salmo 139:14: "Maravillosas son tus obras, y mi alma las conoce muy bien". Tu mente subconsciente controla todas las funciones corporales, ya sea que estés despierto o dormido. Mantiene tu corazón latiendo, tus pulmones respirando y tu sangre oxigenada, con la misma eficacia cuando estás dormido que cuando estás despierto.

Considera la notable historia de un hombre cuya mente subconsciente actuó como una película, con su imagen mental de curación arraigada a través de semanas de pensamiento concentrado. Un día, cuando su teléfono sonó mientras su esposa y enfermera estaban fuera, logró responder a pesar de que estaba a 12 pies de distancia. Ese fue el momento de su curación. Al concentrarse en el poder curativo de su mente subconsciente, lo activó, lo que le permitió caminar a pesar de que anteriormente creía que no podía.

Esto ilustra La profunda influencia de la mente subconsciente. Se la puede comparar con un depósito oculto de poder curativo, que muchas personas han creído que existe en su interior durante siglos. Los relatos históricos de diversas culturas sugieren que los antiguos sacerdotes y hombres santos ejercían este poder, invocándolo a través de oraciones, rituales y diversos símbolos para lograr la curación. Dichas prácticas variaban ampliamente: algunas implicaban la imposición de manos, mientras que otras utilizaban amuletos, talismanes o conjuros.

Incluso hoy, su mente subconsciente está trabajando continuamente, regulando funciones corporales esenciales ya sea que esté despierto o dormido. Por ejemplo, su corazón late rítmicamente y sus pulmones mantienen su función sin esfuerzo consciente. Su mente subconsciente también supervisa procesos intrincados como la digestión y las secreciones hormonales. Cabe destacar que mientras duerme, su cuerpo continúa con funciones vitales como el crecimiento del cabello y la secreción de sudor, y se han hecho muchos grandes descubrimientos en los sueños.

Sin embargo, las emociones negativas como la preocupación, la ansiedad y la tristeza pueden alterar el ritmo natural de los sistemas de su cuerpo. Para restablecer la armonía, es esencial calmar la mente y dejar que el subconsciente tome el control de una manera pacífica y ordenada. Comuníquese con su mente subconsciente con convicción y ella responderá en consecuencia, esforzándose por mantener su bienestar.

Su mente subconsciente está intrínsecamente diseñada para mantenerlo vivo y saludable. Manifiesta instintos protectores, como hacer que vomite si ingiere algo dañino. Cuando confía en su poder milagroso, trabaja para restaurar su salud.

Para aprovechar este poder de manera efectiva, primero comprenda que su subconsciente siempre está activo, operando las 24 horas del día independientemente de su conciencia. Su mente consciente necesita concentrarse en pensamientos positivos y constructivos. Al mantener su mente consciente ocupada con expectativas alentadoras, permite que su subconsciente genere resultados beneficiosos.

Considere el principio curativo observado en la historia de una mujer de Francia que recuperó la vista a pesar de tener nervios ópticos sin vida. Este evento milagroso, relatado por Ruth Cranston en la revista McCall, subraya cómo la creencia y la fe en la mente subconsciente pueden producir curación. La recuperación de la vista de Madame no se debió a factores externos, sino más bien a la respuesta de su mente subconsciente a su fe.

De manera similar, en Johannesburgo, un predicador protestante utilizó una técnica para visualizar una salud perfecta, afirmándola con una relajación profunda y creencias positivas. Este método condujo a una recuperación notable de la leucemia. Otro ejemplo involucró a un hombre con parálisis funcional que se visualizó caminando y realizando actividades diarias. Su mente subconsciente aceptó esta imagen mental y lo ayudó a recuperar la salud.

Históricamente, varias prácticas curativas implicaban sugestiones hipnóticas y rituales para involucrar a la mente subconsciente, lo que condujo a recuperaciones notables. Estas prácticas revelan que el poder de la mente subconsciente, cuando se alinea con la fe y la creencia, puede efectuar cambios significativos.

La perspectiva bíblica refuerza este concepto. Como se menciona en la Biblia, "Todo lo que pidas en la oración, cree que lo has recibido, y lo tendrás". Este principio sugiere que para manifestar tus deseos, debes creer y aceptar plenamente que tu deseo ya se ha cumplido. La fe juega un papel crucial, ya que la mente debe visualizar el resultado deseado como una realidad para que se haga realidad. Esta creencia debe estar profundamente arraigada en su subconsciente, nutriéndola como una semilla que crecerá hasta convertirse en realidad.

Al centrar sus pensamientos en resultados positivos y reforzarlos con una fe inquebrantable, puede aprovechar el poder creativo de su mente subconsciente, convirtiendo sus metas y deseos en realidad. Así como las semillas se convierten en plantas con el cuidado adecuado, sus creencias y expectativas dan forma a las experiencias de su vida.

Puede aprovechar el poder creativo de su mente siguiendo estos pasos. En el mundo del subconsciente, sus pensamientos, ideas, planes y metas se vuelven reales, al igual que las partes de su cuerpo físico. El método bíblico para lograrlo implica eliminar cualquier condición o evento que pueda sugerir un fracaso. Al plantar una idea o meta positiva en su mente subconsciente y dejarla intacta, crecerá hasta convertirse en realidad. La fe es crucial aquí; es similar a creer que las semillas que planta se convertirán en plantas porque confía en las reglas del crecimiento y la agricultura.

La Biblia enfatiza la fe como una forma de pensar, un estado mental y una certeza interior de que el pensamiento que acepta se manifestará en la realidad. La fe implica confiar en lo que puede parecer improbable o imposible para la mente consciente y entregarse al poder del subconsciente. Esto significa dejar de lado el escepticismo lógico y abrazar plenamente el potencial de su mente subconsciente para lograr cambios.

Los milagros en los santuarios de todo el mundo ofrecen evidencia convincente de este principio. En Japón, por ejemplo, la gente visita el famoso santuario del Gran Buda, un templo de 42Estatua de bronce de 1,5 metros de alto conocida por su postura meditativa. Los visitantes hacen ofrendas, encienden velas y expresan sus súplicas. Una jovencita, después de rezar y hacer ofrendas, recuperó la voz, un acontecimiento milagroso que atribuyó a la intervención de Buda. Su fe y su ritual crearon un estado mental que permitió que su mente subconsciente respondiera y la sanara.

Consideremos la historia de un familiar con cáncer cuya recuperación ilustra el poder de la fe y la imaginación. Su hijo, que creía profundamente en el poder curativo de una reliquia, fabricó un trozo de madera para que pareciera un artefacto sagrado. Cuando su padre lo sostuvo, rezó y se durmió, su condición mejoró notablemente. La verdadera curación provino de su fe y su imaginación despiertas, no de la reliquia en sí.

Esto demuestra un principio curativo universal: independientemente del método o la tradición, el poder subyacente es la mente subconsciente. Diferentes prácticas curativas, desde la osteopatía y la quiropráctica hasta varios rituales religiosos, se basan en este único proceso. La fe juega un papel vital; desencadena las capacidades curativas de la mente subconsciente. Las investigaciones sobre la hipnosis demuestran que la mente subconsciente puede influir significativamente en las funciones corporales. Por ejemplo, una persona bajo hipnosis puede presentar síntomas como fiebre alta o escalofríos basándose únicamente en sugestiones. De manera similar, un sujeto hipnótico puede desarrollar reacciones alérgicas u otras afecciones simplemente a través de la sugestión, lo que pone de relieve que la influencia de la mente se extiende a la salud física.

También se producen curaciones notables mediante otras formas de terapia, como la osteopatía y los métodos quiroprácticos, que demuestran el mismo principio: la mente subconsciente como sanador principal. Los procesos naturales de curación del cuerpo, como curar un corte, dependen de la capacidad de la mente subconsciente para mantener y restaurar la salud.

Personajes históricos como Paracelso, un alquimista y cirujano suizo, reconocieron el poder de la fe en la curación. Afirmó que, independientemente de que la fe se deposite en un objeto genuino o falso, los resultados serán los mismos. Esta opinión fue compartida por otros pensadores que vieron los efectos de la fe y la imaginación como fundamentales para la curación.

En los tiempos modernos, ejemplos como los experimentos del Dr. Bernheim con terapias sugestivas ilustran aún más el poder de la mente subconsciente. Mediante la aplicación de sugestiones sencillas, podía inducir síntomas o incluso causar cambios físicos, lo que reforzaba la idea de que la mente subconsciente gobierna nuestro estado físico.

El principio sigue siendo claro: la mente subconsciente es fundamental para toda curación. Ya sea a través de la fe, la imaginación o la sugestión, el verdadero poder reside en la profundidad con la que interactuamos con nuestras creencias y expectativas subconscientes.

Queridos amigos y familiares,

Al sentarme a escribir esta carta, me siento abrumado por la gratitud que siento por cada uno de ustedes. Su apoyo inquebrantable, su aliento y su fe en mí han sido simplemente increíbles. Ya sea animándome desde la distancia, ofreciéndome palabras de sabiduría o simplemente estando ahí para escucharme, su presencia en mi vida ha marcado toda la diferencia.

Escribir a menudo se considera una actividad solitaria, pero su apoyo me ha demostrado que, en realidad, se necesita una comunidad. Han celebrado mis éxitos y me han levantado en momentos de duda. Su creencia en el panorama general, en mis sueños y aspiraciones, ha sido una fuente constante de motivación.

No se trata solo de las palabras en la página; se trata del viaje que hemos recorrido juntos. Cada uno de ustedes ha jugado un papel único en la formación de quien soy como escritor y como persona. Sus ideas, amor y apoyo incondicional me han inspirado a seguir adelante, incluso cuando el camino parecía incierto.

Gracias por creer en mí, incluso cuando yo mismo dudaba de mí. Gracias por comprender los sacrificios que conlleva perseguir un sueño. Gracias por su paciencia, su comprensión y su interminable aliento.

A medida que continúo en este viaje, sepan que llevo a cada uno de ustedes en mi corazón. Su apoyo no solo me ha ayudado a alcanzar mis metas, sino que también ha enriquecido mi vida de maneras que no puedo expresar plenamente. Me siento verdaderamente bendecido por tener amigos y familiares tan increíbles a mi lado.

Con la más profunda gratitud y amor,

Una Oración de Gratitud

Padre Celestial, Creador de todo lo visible e invisible, me presento ante Ti con un corazón rebosante de gratitud. Las palabras parecen insuficientes para expresar la profundidad de mi agradecimiento, pero las ofrezco con sinceridad, sabiendo que comprendes incluso los susurros más silenciosos de mi alma.

Gracias, Señor, por el aliento en mis pulmones, los latidos de mi corazón y la vida que me has concedido con tanta gracia. Cada momento en que despierto es un testimonio de Tu misericordia, y cada paso que doy está guiado por Tu insondable sabiduría. Estoy asombrado de Tu creación: la belleza del mundo que me rodea, las complejidades de la vida y el asombro de la existencia. Cada amanecer me recuerda Tu fidelidad, y cada noche estrellada, Tu infinita majestad.

Te doy gracias por los desafíos y las pruebas que me han moldeado, porque sé que en cada dificultad hay una lección, y en cada tristeza, una comprensión más profunda de Tu amor. Has sido mi fortaleza cuando estaba débil, mi consuelo en tiempos de desesperación y mi luz en los días más oscuros. Incluso cuando no podía ver el camino por delante, Tú estabas allí, guiándome con un amor que no conoce límites.

Gracias por las bendiciones que a menudo doy por sentadas: el calor de un hogar, el abrazo de los seres queridos, el alimento que nutre mi cuerpo y la paz que calma mi espíritu. Estoy agradecido por las personas que has puesto en mi vida, cada una de ellas un reflejo de Tu amor y un recordatorio de la comunidad que has tejido a mi alrededor. Que sientan Tu presencia como yo la siento, y que sean bendecidos abundantemente por la bondad y el amor que me han mostrado.

Señor, te agradezco por Tu Palabra, una fuente de sabiduría, guía y consuelo. En sus páginas encuentro la fuerza para perseverar, el valor para enfrentar mis miedos y la certeza de que nunca estoy solo. Tus promesas son mi ancla, y Tu verdad es mi fundamento.

Al ofrecer esta oración de agradecimiento, humildemente pido Tus bendiciones para todos los que lean estas palabras. Que sientan Tu amor rodeándolos, llenando sus corazones de paz y sus vidas de alegría. Que encuentren fuerza en Tu presencia, consuelo en Tus promesas y esperanza en el conocimiento de que siempre estás con ellos.

Bendícelos, Señor, con la abundancia de Tu gracia. Concédeles sabiduría en sus decisiones, paz en sus corazones y gozo en su camino. Que Tu luz guíe sus pasos, y que Tu amor sea un recordatorio constante de la bondad que proviene de caminar en Tus caminos.

Padre, te elevo todos los deseos de mi corazón, expresados y no expresados, sabiendo que Tú escuchas y respondes de maneras que están más allá de mi comprensión. Confío en Tu tiempo, Tu voluntad y Tu bondad infinita.

Con cada aliento, te doy gracias. Con cada pensamiento, alabo Tu nombre. Que mi vida sea un reflejo de la gratitud que siento, y que todo lo que haga glorifique a Ti, el Altísimo, ahora y siempre.

En Tu santo nombre, te lo pido.

Amén.

www.ingramcontent.com/pod-product-compliance
Lightning Source LLC
Chambersburg PA
CBHW071555260726